Sue wrote: Well thought out presentation of EFT and Anxiety

Having 80 tapping statements that address many, many aspects of anxiety and worry is really helpful. Following each group of statements, there is a space for journaling. This helps to retrieve memories facilitating the effectiveness of the tapping.

Tessa gives definitions of anxiety and worry that aid the reader in increasing self awareness of the possible drivers behind behaviors, other mood states, and other emotions. This aids in broadening the number of possible targets to use Tapping on which ensures thorough treatment and good results.

Very helpful and well thought out presentation of EFT and Anxiety.

Nick H. wrote: Very Powerful Book!

I have had the great privilege of working with Tessa Cason and have experienced the true life changing power in her Presence, in her words, and in her books. After tapping just a few of these statements, I went from feeling low energy and depressed to feeling a peace and love that I had not felt for quite some time. She is a remarkable person and an extremely gifted healer, counselor, and writer.

Reading this book and tapping these statements will change your life. It changed mine. Thank you Tessa!

Corrine Hill wrote: Excellent

I am new to tapping and have had some powerful experiences. I find this helpful to those who like me have trouble with what to say. I highly recommend this book to everyone. Grateful!

Gnostic View wrote: Excellent Techniques from a Master Teacher

Tessa is a gifted and compassionate teacher and coach. I can't think of anyone who would not benefit from time spent with her or with her writings. EFT works. You can learn from one of the best, and these short but precise books are a great way to move ahead with EFT.

Lshep wrote: Great Book!

Another extremely helpful and well written book by Tessa Cason! I really appreciate the stories and found that the statements really resonated with me. Easy to understand and follow. I am so grateful for her EFT books!

39428 wrote: Very Helpful!

What an excellent tapping statement book! The book is arranged well. It leads tappers through an easy-to-relate to story, a description of how anxiety and worry affects our life, EFT basics for those new to EFT, and then the gold, the tapping statements.

There's a nice variety of relevant tapping statements offered which allows readers to go as deeply as they want into this work. Love the quotes throughout the book too. The positive statements are a nice way to end.

I highly recommend this book! Thank you, Tessa.

Amazon Customer wrote: Future helps present

I was a bit unsure about this as it is not something that I would usually look at. With the persuasion of my wife we started the journey. I must admit, it was quietly surprised. Once we tried it a few times I noticed that it began to make a difference.

New book releases are free the first 24 hours. To know of new releases and dates for free downloads, please subscribe at www.TessaCason.com

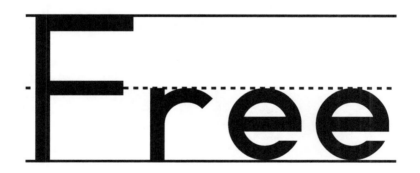

80 EFT Tapping Statements™ for Anxiety and Worry

Includes a Bonus of 60 Tapping Statements

Tessa Cason, MA

Tessa Cason
5694 Mission Ctr. Rd. #602-213
San Diego, CA. 92108
www.TessaCason.com
Tessa@TessaCason.com

LEGAL NOTICE AND DISCLAIMER:

From author and publisher: The information in this book is not intended to diagnose or treat any particular disease and/or condition. Nothing contained herein is meant to replace qualified medical or psychological advice and/or services. The author and publisher do not assume responsibility for how the reader chooses to apply the techniques herein. Use of the information is at the reader's discretion and discernment. The author and publisher specifically disclaim any and all liability arising directly or indirectly from the use or application contained in this book.

Nothing contained in this book is to be considered medical advice for any specific situation. This information is not intended as a substitute for the advice or medical care of a physician prior to taking any personal action with respect to the information contained in this book. This book and all of its contents are intended for educational and informational purposes only. The information in this book is believed to be reliable, but is presented without guaranty or warranty.

By reading further, you agree to release the author and publisher from any damages or injury associated with your use of the material in this book.

Table of Contents

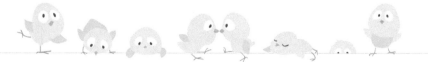

My EFT Tapping Story

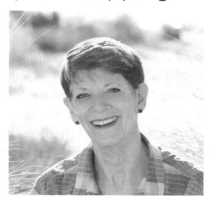

I watched from the audience as the musical group, The 5th Dimension, sang their song, "Age of Aquarius, Let the Sunshine In." In 1970, this song soared to the top of the charts. *Age of Aquarius,* I thought. *What does that mean?*

In 1970, I couldn't do a Google search for "Age of Aquarius." There weren't any websites or blogs I could read to find information about the "dawning of a new age." There weren't any YouTube videos to watch. The internet didn't exist in 1970. We had books, audiobooks on cassette tapes, and occasionally, a live, in-person seminar.

Another "new age" seeker, Cindy, and I searched for self-help, self-improvement, spiritual, and personal development classes, books, audiobooks, basically anything that could increase our awareness of the new age that was dawning.

Cindy was friends with a woman named Donna Eden. Donna had just returned from a workshop about energy. When we asked if she would teach us what was taught in the workshop, she agreed. One afternoon, a small group of us sat on her living room floor as Donna conducted her own mini workshop for us. Part of our mini workshop included how to muscle-test, a technique used to ask the body questions that bypass the conscious mind.

"Cindy, have you heard of a woman named Louise Hay?" I asked. "She is leading a workshop in La Jolla to help those with AIDS." Cindy and I attended. Louise believed that our thoughts influenced our health. In the 1970s, people didn't believe the food they ate impacted their health. The concept that our thoughts could impact our health was revolutionary for the time!

Knowing I was searching for answers on how to heal my dysfunctional childhood, Cindy suggested the "Fischer-Hoffman Process, Getting a Loving Divorce from Mom and Dad." She had just completed the program. Cindy neglected to mention the time-consuming homework, about thirty hours, every weekend for thirteen weeks! I did complete the exhausting, but liberating program.

The facilitators for the process hosted a weekly gathering in their home for Siddha Yoga and guru Swami Muktananda, the father of Siddha Yoga. After completing the program, I flew to New York and drove to the Catskills in upstate New York. I lived in the ashram for two months taking classes about Siddha Yoga, the self, and self-realization. Muktananda was in residence for a month while I was there. I attended his nightly meeting.

My journey for personal growth led to Murrieta Hot Springs in Southern California. A group called *Alive Polarity* offered workshops to transform the self. Students lived at the retreat while attending their workshops. I completed two workshops, living at the retreat for fourteen weeks. We met six days a week, six to seven hours each day. It was as intense as going through boot camp.

I learned the value of Gestalt therapy and the "empty chair technique." Gestalt therapy is a form of psychotherapy that views each individual as a blend of the mind, emotions, body, and soul with unique experiences and realities. The "empty chair technique" is used to address unresolved issues, conflicts, and emotions.

In 1985, a new breakfast group was formed called The Inside Edge. We met once a week at 6 AM for breakfast and a speaker. I heard new authors such as Brian Tracy, Jack Canfield, Mark Victor Hansen, Susan Jeffers, and many others after they had written their first books.

At this time, I was employed at The Learning Annex, assisting with hosting events. The Learning Annex was an education company that offered a wide range of classes with diverse topics. This is a short list of speakers I heard speak:

* Wayne Dyer
* James Redfield
* Dan Millman
* David Hawkins
* Deepak Chopra
* Marianne Williamson
* Melody Beattie

* Neale Donald Walsch
* Byron Katie
* Don Miguel Ruiz
* Richard Bach

In 1988, I attended a promo event for a new speaker on the lecture circuit, Tony Robbins. I returned for the weekend event, which included a firewalk. Without the internet in 1988, there were no YouTube videos or internet searches to prepare oneself for Tony or for walking on fire. Saying that *UPW, Unleash the Power Within*, was the most transformational event I have ever completed falls short of how spectacular and life changing UPW was.

The three-day event began on Friday. Throughout the first day, Tony had us do various exercises to prepare us for the firewalk. Around midnight, he marched the entire room of people to the parking lot.

As we approached the asphalt, we heard tribal drums beating, the crackling of logs burning, and smelled the burning embers. When the huge pile of wood came into view, we felt the blast of heat coming off the fire. Flames and sparks were shooting high into the air. The immediate thought one has is *Really? I am going to walk across that? That's fire. It's hot and it burns!*

Around 3 AM, everyone in the ballroom once again marched to the parking lot. We found rows of embers, ten feet long, with staff at each line. With the drums beating, excitement in the air, and everyone chanting, we lined up behind a row of coals.

When we reached the front of the line, a staff member determined if we were truly ready. They looked us in the eye, assessed our psychological readiness, looked at our body language, and told us to either go or to get back in line because we were not ready.

At the end of the bed of coals, our feet were sprayed with cool water, and then someone was there to celebrate with us. It was an amazing experience. Thirty-five years later, I still remember walking across red-hot coals and feeling triumphant as I celebrated the achievement.

In 1988, I completed every program and event Tony had, which included Date with Destiny and Mastery University. After attending all the programs, I volunteered to staff his events and helped with a dozen fire walks.

At Mastery Universe, Tony had a thirty-five-foot firewalk along with the ten-foot bed of coals. After confidently walking the ten-foot bed of coals, I walked the thirty-five-foot, and then went back and did the ten-foot bed of coals again. It was fun!

After attending numerous trainings, and earning various certificates and degrees, I established a life coaching practice in 1996, when life coaching was in its infancy. After several years, I realized that desire, exploration, and awareness did not equate to change and transformation for my clients.

Exploring the underlying cause of their pain, knowing their motivation to change, and defining who they wanted to become, did not create the changes in their lives they desired.

My livelihood depended on the success of my clients. I realized I needed a tool, technique, or method to aid my clients in their quest for change.

At the time, I knew that everything in our lives, all of our thoughts and feelings, choices and decisions, habits and experiences, actions and reactions, were the result of our beliefs.

I knew that the beliefs were "stored" in our subconscious mind.

I knew to transform and change our lives, we needed to heal the underlying unhealthy, dysfunctional beliefs on the subconscious level. I needed a tool, technique, or method to eliminate and heal the unhealthy beliefs stored in the subconscious mind.

I visited a friend who managed a bookstore and told her of my dilemma, that I needed something to help my clients truly change and transform their lives. She reached for a book on the counter near the register. "People have been raving about this book on EFT, Emotional Freedom Technique. Try it and see if it can help your clients."

In the 1990s, the internet was not an everyday part of our lives. Popular books sold more by word of mouth than by any other means. Managing a bookstore, my friend knew what worked and what did not work. I trusted my friend, so I purchased the book.

As I read the book and discovered that EFT was tapping our heads, I was unsure if this was the technique that would help my clients. I had some adventurous and forgiving clients whom I taught how to tap. When **every single client** returned for their next appointment and shared how different their lives had been that week because of tapping, I took notice! I was intrigued.

I learned that the first statement we needed to tap was: "It's not okay or safe for my life to change."

I learned that clearing an emotional memory was different from clearing beliefs.

I learned that for EFT Tapping to work, we needed to find the underlying cause of an issue.

Have you heard the joke about the drunk looking for his keys under a street lamp? A policeman asks the man what he is looking for. "My keys," says the drunk. The policeman joins in the search. Not finding the keys, the policeman asks the drunk if this is where he lost his keys.

"No, I lost them in the park."

Confused, the policeman says, "Why are you looking here and not over there?"

The drunk answers, "The light is brighter here."

EFT Tapping is a simple, yet highly effective tool to heal our issues by addressing the cause and not just the symptoms. Addressing the symptoms would be like looking for the keys under the street light. The symptoms are easily identified. But, healing the symptoms does not heal the underlying cause.

I learned we are complex, complicated beings wrapped up with a lot of history, traumas, dramas, and experiences. Sometimes finding the cause is like walking through a maze...there are a lot of dead ends, turns, and wandering around aimlessly.

Clients started asking for tapping homework. I wrote out statements for them to tap. Soon, I had a library of tapping statements on different emotional issues.

I have been an EFT Practitioner since 2000. Working with hundreds of clients, one-on-one, I learned how to successfully utilize EFT so my clients could grow and transform their lives.

Chapter 1
Introduction

The truth is that our finest moments are most likely
to occur when we are feeling deeply uncomfortable,
unhappy, or unfulfilled. For it is only in such moments,
propelled by our discomfort, that we are likely to
step out of our ruts and start searching
for different ways or truer answers.

M. Scott Peck

Anxiety is an internal response to a perceived threat to our well-being. We feel threatened by an abstract, unknown danger that could harm us in the future.

Worry is a mild form of anxiety. Worry is a tendency to mull anxiety-provoking thoughts over and over. It is thinking, in an obsessive way, about something that has happened or might happen and asking, "What should I have done? What will I do?"

Anxiety is a combination of 4 things:
unidentified Anger, Hurt, Fear, and Self Pity.

Two anxiety-driven behaviors are overcompensating and avoidance. With overcompensating, we are trying to reduce the anxiety, whereas with avoidance, we are trying to escape or avoid the situation that is causing the anxiety. The most common form of avoidance is procrastination.

What we focus on expands.

Anxiety can lead to:
* distrust, emotional withdrawal, and distancing
* hopelessness and low self-esteem
* addictions, alcoholism, and eating disorders
* anger and violence
* workaholism and the need to be super-human
* being overly concerned for others and emotional dependence

Some of the mental symptoms of anxiety include helplessness, confusion, apprehension, negative and/or jumbled thoughts racing through our mind, and feeling that everything is spinning out of control.

The physical symptoms range from muscle tension to a pounding heart, sinking feeling in the stomach, nausea, terrifying feelings of impending doom, sensation of suffocation, flush of heat and sweat alternating with freezing paralysis, shallow breathing, and increased blood pressure.

Anxiety and stress are slightly different. Anxiety is associated with a vague threat, whereas stress is a feeling of being over-whelmed.

With anxiety, our thoughts lean toward the worst-case scenario. With stress, our thoughts are dulled from the fatigue.

With anxiety, we feel revved-up, nervous, tense, on edge, and jumpy, whereas with stress, we feel exhausted, sad, depressed, resentful, and/or moody.

There is something we can do to eliminate the worry and anxiety. It is called EFT Tapping, Emotional Freedom Technique.

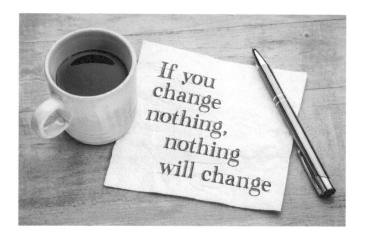

Chapter 2
Mary's Story

"Mary, I can't do this anymore," Frank says. "Your worry and anxiety are just too much for me."

As tears well up in Mary's eyes, she asks Frank, her husband of twelve years, "What are you saying? That our marriage is over? You want a divorce?"

"I just can't do this anymore. You worry about everything. When we got married, your anxiety was something that you had every now and then. Now, you are paranoid about everything. I leave for work, and you act like you are never going to see me again. Either I'm going to be killed, or I'm having an affair.

"I'm not having an affair, but I am constantly being accused of one. That's not me. I am faithful. I have been since the day we met. But now, I am constantly on trial for sins that I haven't even committed."

"I am so sorry Frank," whispers Mary.

"You accused me again last night of having an affair when I got hung up in traffic. I come home straight from work, so you don't think I'm out meeting other women. I stopped playing golf with my friends because you thought I was meeting other women. I have done everything to alleviate your concerns. I've stopped living my life because of your fears and anxiety."

Mary wants to approach Frank yet knows it is not the right thing to do. She doesn't know what to say. Mary continues to sit on the couch, looking down at her hands as they twist in her lap. She can't hold back the tears any longer, as they begin rolling down her cheeks. In a whisper, Mary asks, "Do you want a divorce?"

Frank sits down on the couch next to Mary, taking her hands in his. "I don't know, Mary. I can't live my life, every second of every day, trying to soothe your anxieties. I have stopped being me and that doesn't feel good any longer. Every year, your anxiety and worrying get worse, not better. If you can't get a handle on your anxiety, I can't live with you."

From Frank's last sentence, Mary feels a little bit of hope. He didn't say the D-word. Maybe she has some time to get a handle on the anxiety. She wants to. Her anxiety is even driving her nuts.

As soon as Frank leaves for work, Mary calls one of her best friends and asks for the name of a therapist. Once she hangs up, Mary calls the therapist and schedules an appointment.
Upon meeting Dr. Davidson for the first time, Mary can't speak when he asks why she has come to see him. She chokes back tears, unable to say anything.

Dr. Davidson hands Mary a box of tissues and waits until she is able to speak.

"My husband, Frank, we've been married twelve years, doesn't want to deal with my anxiety any longer. I'm here to see if I can get a handle on it. That's what he wants."

Dr. Davidson asks, "That's what Frank wants. What do you want? Do you want to get a handle on your anxiety?"

"Oh, yes," responds Mary in a near whisper. "I love Frank with all my heart. I don't want to lose him. He's the best thing that ever happened to me."

"Tell me about the anxiety, Mary," says Dr. Davidson with a gentle, understanding voice.

"I tend to mull things over and over in my mind. Soon, the molehill has become a mountain, and I'm convinced the mountain is real, even though I know it isn't. But I am sure that it is!"

"Can you give me an example?"

"Well, last night Frank was late getting home. He said he was stuck in traffic, but I was convinced that he stopped to see a woman. He said he has been faithful since the day we met."

"Do you believe him?"

"Yes, I do. I know Frank isn't having an affair, but I just can't stop thinking about it. What would I do if I found out that he was having an affair? What does she have that I don't? What would I do if Frank and I divorced? Where would I live? How would I pay the bills?"

"Has your anxiety always been so overwhelming?"

"No, it hasn't. Over the years, my anxiety has gotten worse. Now, I'm anxious about almost everything. I can't seem to stop.

"I focus on the worst-case scenario. I get nervous, tense, and feel on edge. My stomach feels queasy, my palms sweat, and my heart races. My thoughts get jumbled, I am apprehensive, and I end up confused. I don't trust myself. I don't trust Frank. I don't trust anything or anyone. Everything feels hopeless."

Dr. Davidson explains, "Anxiety is a combination of four things: unidentified anger, hurt, fear, and self-pity. Can you relate to any of these four things?"

Mary sits back in her chair and ponders. "I get angry that I go over and over the 'what ifs.' What if Frank has an affair? What if Frank and I divorce? What if this is really the end of my marriage? I don't have any control over my thoughts. It feels like my world is spinning out of control."

"Mary," Dr. Davidson asks, "are you willing to deal with your anxiety?"

"If you had asked me a week ago, I would have told you that I am powerless to live my life any differently. I can't stop worrying, and I am a chronic worrier. I worry that my anxiety and constant worrying are incurable. I have difficulty turning my worry off. I will never be able to let my fears go."

"And now?" Dr. Davidson asks.

"And now," Mary ponders. "Now, I hope that I can stop worrying. I don't want to worry anymore or at all! I want to let my fears go! My anxiety paralyzes me, and I don't want to be powerless any longer. I am controlled by my worry. I torture myself with the worst-case scenarios. I want to torture myself with love and joy.

"I am so tired of turning every error that I make into a catastrophe. I'm tired of being hopeless and helpless. I know that I am my own worst enemy. I know that I focus on the negative instead of the positive. How stupid is that?!"

"Well, I agree. Not so smart."

"Every time that I start to feel good about myself, I am overcome with self-doubt. I get angry at myself for feeling flawed."

"So, you can relate to the anger," says Dr. Davidson. "And the hurt? How has that shown up in your life?"

"I am hurt that my anxiety has been such a huge motivating force in my life. You would think that the love of a fantastic man would compensate for my anxiety. At first, it did," says Mary.

"At first, it did?"

"Over time, the love I felt for Frank paled in comparison to how inferior I felt to others," says Mary with a sigh. "And now, well...the more inferior I feel, the more I worry. The more I worry, the more Frank pulls away. My anxiety is creating the reality that I am trying to prevent. Ironic, don't you think?"

"Frank was a motivation in the beginning?"

"Yes. I love him so much. I still do. But then I start to worry about all the bad things that could happen. The worrisome thoughts recycle endlessly in my mind. There is no space in my mind to think about Frank, his love for me, or the love I have for him."

Dr. Davidson interrupts Mary and asks, "Do you deserve to be successful, happy, and loved, Mary?"

"I think not. I know that I make things worse because of my anxiety. I know that I tend to exaggerate and make the worst-case scenarios worse than they are. I know that Frank isn't having an affair."

"Do you feel that if you worry, it will prevent bad things from happening?"

"As silly as I know it sounds, yes. Even though I know my worrying makes situations worse, I will never learn how to be comfortable in the world. My worry keeps me keyed up and restless," responds Mary.

"I have one last question for you, Mary," says Dr. Davidson. "Do you have the desire and ability to overcome your anxiety?"

Mary takes a deep breath and slowly lets it out. Then another. Desire, I have, she thinks. But ability? How am I to find the ability when I am so mired with pain, struggle, and suffering? How could I ever trust myself to create a joyous life?

Finally, Mary says, "I don't know how, Dr. Davidson. Desire, yes. I want my marriage. But how to overcome the anxiety, I don't know. If I knew how, I would have done it a long time ago."

"I do," responds Dr. Davidson. "I would like to introduce you to a simple, yet highly effective, tool and process called EFT tapping, Emotional Freedom Technique."

Six months later, Dr. Davidson opens his mail to find an invitation to Mary and Frank's ceremony to renew their marriage vows.

Dr. Davidson marvels at Mary's courage during the ceremony. After the ceremony, Mary introduces Frank to Dr. Davidson. With a huge grin on his face, Frank shakes Dr. Davidson's hand. "You are a miracle worker, Dr. Davidson. You gave me back my sweet Mary. She even taught me the tapping thing. When anything comes up, we tap on it together. It has worked wonders in our relationship. Thank you so much!"

Dr. Davidson looks over to see a happy, joyous, beautiful Mary beaming at her husband. He feels a warm fulfillment and satisfaction inside.

Chapter 3
Discovering EFT Tapping

Our behavior, what we do and say, is determined by our beliefs. Beliefs precede all of our actions, reactions, thoughts, feelings, experiences, and habits.

In 2000, Johnnie was one of my life coaching clients. A life coach is someone who works with their clients to identify their goals, and the steps and tasks needed to accomplish their objectives. As much as Johnnie wanted to perform the steps to accomplish his goals, week after week, he was not able to.

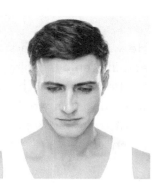

Johnnie's main issue was not feeling good enough about himself. As a result, he withdrew from society, made himself wrong whenever he "messed up," and was a perfectionist.

Johnnie wasn't the only client struggling to fulfill their weekly assignments. I knew underneath the "not feeling good enough" were dysfunctional beliefs and I needed a tool or technique, something, to help my clients move beyond their stumbling blocks.

On a whim, I introduced tapping to Johnnie. I had just finished reading a book on EFT, Emotional Freedom Technique, and was doubtful about its effectiveness. I did not know how tapping one's head would change their life. I did know from what I read that tapping could change dysfunctional beliefs on a subconscious level. I thought, "Nothing ventured, nothing gained."

The following appointment, Johnnie reported back that he had gone to lunch with a group of his fellow employees to celebrate someone's birthday. He had been asked numerous times to accompany them to functions away from the office before, and every time Johnnie declined. He was sure other people saw him as he saw himself, not good enough.

He was amazed. First, that he went to lunch and second, he actually enjoyed himself. He contributed the shift in himself to the tapping. "That's the only thing different between last week and this week," he told me. I was surprised he actually went to lunch, enjoyed himself, and that tapping made a difference.

During that session, Johnnie and I talked about the beliefs that he felt contributed to not feeling good enough and less than others. It was eye-opening for me and shifted the way I conducted sessions.

To change our lives, we need to address the underlying cause of an issue. We need to uncover dysfunctional beliefs, and then, eliminate them from the subconscious.

A belief is accepting something to be true, whether it is Truth or not. A dysfunctional belief is a belief that takes us away from peace, love, joy, stability, acceptance, and harmony. It causes us to feel stressed, fearful, anxious, and/or insecure.

Beliefs are "stored" in the subconscious mind. The subconscious is the part of the mind responsible for all of our involuntary actions, like our heartbeat and breathing rate. It does not evaluate, make decisions, or pass judgment. It just is. It does not determine if something is "right" or "wrong."

The subconscious is much like the software of a computer. Just as a computer can only do what it has been programmed to do, we can only do as we are programmed to do.

Our programming is determined by our beliefs. Beliefs and memories are "stored" in the subconscious.

The conscious mind is the part of us that thinks, passes judgments, makes decisions, remembers, analyzes, has desires, and communicates with others. It is responsible for logic and reasoning, understanding and comprehension. The mind determines our actions, feelings, thoughts, judgments, and decisions based on our beliefs.

EFT TAPPING

EFT Tapping, Emotional Freedom Technique, is a tool that allows us to change dysfunctional beliefs and emotions on a subconscious level. It involves making a statement while tapping different points along traditional Chinese meridian pathways.

The general principle behind EFT is that the cause of all negative emotions is a disruption in the body's energy system. By tapping on locations where several different meridians flow, we can release unproductive memories, emotions, and beliefs that cause the blockages.

After the shift in Johnnie and other clients, I was determined to discover how to utilize EFT Tapping to help other clients effectively eliminate dysfunctional beliefs. After teaching tapping to ten clients, I had all the clients come in for a group session. We called it Discovery Evening and spent a fun evening exploring different aspects of tapping to determine how to maximize results. My livelihood was dependent on the success of my clients and thus, I was motivated to learn the most effective methods.

This book is the result of twenty-plus years of doing private sessions as well as teaching classes on EFT Tapping and training others to be practitioners.

Chapter 4
Meridian Tapping

EFT is sometimes referred to as meridian tapping or energy tapping.

The circulatory system moves blood throughout the body. The nervous system is a vast network of nerves that sends electrical signals throughout the body. And the respiratory system brings air into and out of the lungs. But what about energy? What system is responsible for generating and moving energy in the body? The circulatory system has arteries and veins, the nervous system has nerves, and the respiratory system uses blood to supply air to the cells of the body. But, what about energy?

In Chinese philosophy, energy is called "chi," (also known as qi, prana, and life force in other cultures). Chi flows through our bodies and is impacted by every thought we think, every word we speak, every action we take, and every belief we hold.

Traditional Chinese Medicine, thousands of years ago, mapped out the energy pathways in the physical body. These pathways called meridians. Meridians are pathways in which energy travels throughout the body. Think super highway! Think rivers and streams.

When blood and oxygen are able to flow unobstructed, the body is healthy. If there are any restrictions to blood or oxygen flow, illness will result. When an accident happens on a super highway, the flow of traffic is impacted. When rivers and streams become polluted with debris, water stops flowing.

When energy is able to flow freely, unobstructed, the body is healthy. Dis-ease happens when the energy is blocked. Every breath, emotion, and thought reflects the state and quality of our chi. Energy can become blocked by our thoughts, speech, actions, and beliefs as well as stress, injury, and trauma.

Tapping on different points along the energy pathways has the potential to release blocked energy. This is the principle behind EFT Tapping. EFT Tapping activates points along the meridian pathways to release blockages so that energy flows more freely and health is restored.

Chapter 5
How to Tap

There is a long form and a short form of tapping. At our Discovery Evening, we tapped both forms to determine if one was more successful than the other. There was no difference. Both were effective regardless of the dysfunctional belief or emotion we were exploring. Below are the instructions for tapping the short form of EFT Tapping.

EFT Tapping involves 1) making a statement and 2) tapping.

THE EFT TAPPING STATEMENT WE SAY AS WE TAP

An EFT Tapping Statement has three parts:

Part 1: starts with "**Even though**" followed by

Part 2: a statement which could be the **dysfunctional emotion or belief**, and

Part 3: ends with "I **totally and completely accept myself.**"

A complete statement would be, "**Even though I fear change, I totally and completely accept myself.**"

TAPPING INSTRUCTIONS

There are two different segments of the tapping. The first is called "the setup," and the second is the tapping. The following instructions are for the right hand. Reverse the directions to tap using the left hand. It is more effective, to tap only one side rather than both sides simultaneously.

I. SETUP

A. With the fingertips of the right hand, find a tender spot below the left collarbone. Once the tender spot is identified, press firmly on the spot, moving the fingertips in a clockwise, circular motion.

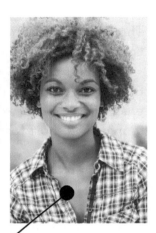

Tender spot below the left collarbone

B. As the fingers circle and press against the tender spot, repeat the tapping statement three times: "Even though, [tapping statement]____, I totally and completely accept myself."

> An example would be: "Even though I fear change, I totally and completely accept myself."

II. TAPPING

A. After repeating the statement three times, tap the following eight points, repeating the [tapping statement] at each point. Tap each point five – ten times:

1. The inner edge of the eyebrow, just above the eye. [I fear change.]
2. Temple, just to the side of the eye. [I fear change.]
3. Just below the eye (on the cheekbone). [I fear change.]
4. Under the nose. [I fear change.]
5. Under the lips. [I fear change.]
6. Under the knob of the collar bone. [I fear change.]
7. Three inches under the arm pit. [I fear change.]
8. Top back of the head. [I fear change.]

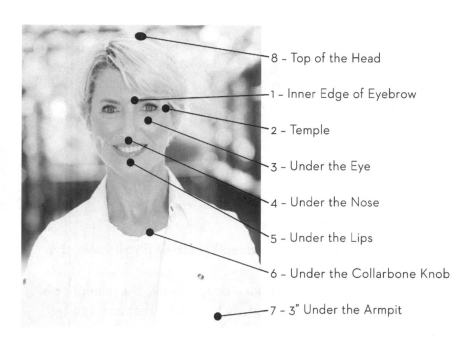

8 – Top of the Head

1 – Inner Edge of Eyebrow

2 – Temple

3 – Under the Eye

4 – Under the Nose

5 – Under the Lips

6 – Under the Collarbone Knob

7 – 3" Under the Armpit

B. After tapping, take a deep breath. If you are not able to take a deep, full, satisfying breath, do eye rolls.

III. EYE ROLLS

A. With one hand, tap continuously on the back of the other hand between the fourth and fifth fingers.
B. Hold your head straight forward, eyes looking straight down.
C. For six seconds, roll your eyes from the floor straight up toward the ceiling while repeating the tapping statement. Keep your head straight forward, only moving your eyes.

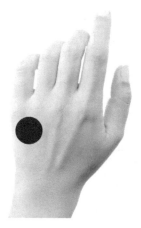

IV. TAKE A DEEP BREATH

A. If you are able to take a deep breath or if you yawn, the statement cleared.
B. If you are not able to take a deep breath, there might be other dysfunctional beliefs or emotions that need to be addressed as well.

ALTERNATIVE TO TAPPING

An alternative to tapping the eight points is to tap the side of the hand, also known as the karate chop point.

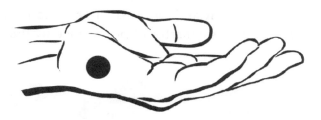

I TOTALLY AND COMPLETELY ACCEPT MYSELF OR I TOTALLY AND COMPLETELY LOVE AND ACCEPT MYSELF.

At the end of the tapping statement, we say: "I totally and completely accept myself." Some practitioners include "love myself." What the Discovery group learned is not everyone loves themselves, and it was difficult for some to make the statement. They paused and cringed every time they said, "I totally and completely love myself."

One client said, "I just can't say that because I know it isn't true. Every time I say, 'I love myself,' I am reminded that I don't and then feel guilty that I don't, and maybe the tapping won't work because I am lying to myself. I can accept myself, but in terms of loving myself, I'm not there yet."

I took notice when others said they felt the same way. For tapping to be most effective, it was best for some to say, "I totally and completely accept myself," rather than, "I totally and completely love and accept myself." The majority of the Discovery

Evening group preferred to leave love out of the statement, so the statement they said was, "I totally and completely accept myself."

The last part of the statement, whether that is "I totally and completely accept myself" or "I totally and completely love and accept myself," is a matter of preference by the tapper.

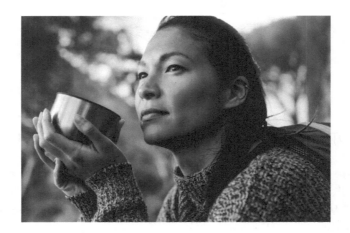

Chapter 6
What We Say as We Tap Is VERY Important!

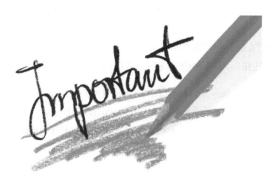

Before the explanation of how and why tapping works, there are several other aspects of tapping that I would like to discuss. One aspect is the tapping statement.

During our Discovery Evening, we experimented with different tapping statements and were able to determine which tapping statements were most effective.

All of our beliefs are programmed into our subconscious minds. If we want to change our lives, we must delete dysfunctional beliefs and emotions on a subconscious level. The statements we say as we tap are the instructions for the subconscious mind and need to be stated in such a way that the unhealthy belief or emotions will be eliminated.

The tapping statements we say as we tap are critical.

Example: You get in a taxi. Several hours later, you still have not arrived at your destination. "*Why?*" you ask. Because you did not give the destination to the taxi driver!

Tapping without an adequate tapping statement is like riding in a cab without giving the cab driver our destination!

TWO CRITICAL ASPECTS OF THE TAPPING STATEMENT

1. TAPPING STATEMENTS THAT AGREE WITH THE CURRENT DYSFUNCTIONAL BELIEF ARE MOST EFFECTIVE.

If the statement we verbalize as we tap does not agree with the current dysfunctional belief, we could end up sabotaging the tapping by forgetting the statement or with other distractions.

For example, you don't feel empowered. You feel like a coward, a failure, and a wimp. If the tapping statement is "I am empowered," the body will remind you that you aren't powerful and not only are you not powerful, but you are also a coward, a failure, and a wimp. If, instead, we tap, "I am not powerful," this statement agrees with the current dysfunctional belief.

The body is less likely to sabotage an EFT Tapping statement that agrees with the current belief.

During the Discovery Evening, as one client was tapping, he stopped in the middle of tapping and said, "It's raining outside." It had been raining all day. It didn't just start raining. This tapper was totally distracted by the rain. The group chuckled, and a discussion followed. We realized the tapping statement needed to agree with the current dysfunctional belief, memory, or emotion to be effective.

The body is here to protect us based on our beliefs, functional or dysfunctional. If the current belief is "I am not powerful," if we were to tap, "I am powerful," the body knows this to not be true and thus, could distract us or sabotage the tapping in some way. The body is less likely to sabotage the tapping and the process if the EFT Tapping statement agrees with the current belief.

2. SUBCONSCIOUS MIND AND TAPPING STATEMENTS

The middle section of the tapping statements are instructions for the subconscious mind. When tapping, we only care what the subconscious hears. There are three rules of the subconscious mind that I like. "The three P Rules."

THREE RULES OF THE SUBCONSCIOUS MIND

1. Personal. It only understands "I," "me," "myself." First-person.

2. Positive. The subconscious does not hear the word "no." When you say, "I am not going to eat that piece of cake," the subconscious hears, "Yummm! Cake! I am going to eat a piece of that cake!"

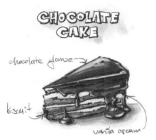

3. Present time. Time does not exist for the subconscious. The only time it knows is "now," present time. "I'm going to clean the garage tomorrow." Tomorrow never comes thus, we constantly put off cleaning the garage.

We tried different types of tapping statements at the Discovery Evening. As my clients were tapping, "I am powerful," many of them found their minds wandering and distracted so much so they forgot what they were tapping.

When we added the word "not" to the tapping statement, "I am not powerful," there were a lot of yawns. A yawn is a signal from the body that a tapping statement cleared. We continued with more statements and added a "no" or "not" to the statement and had tremendous results.

When the statement is "I am not powerful," the **"not"** appeases the physical body, and the subconscious hears, "I am powerful!" Now, my clients only want to tap statements that include a "no" or "not" in the statements. They think tapping statements with a "no" or "not" are brilliant. I agree.

As tappers, we only care what the subconscious hears. It does not hear the word "no."

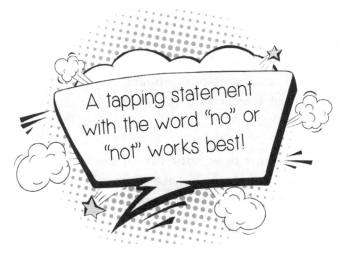

A tapping statement with the word "no" or "not" works best!

Chapter 7
Pattern Interrupt

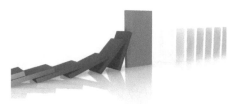

Another topic I want to discuss before moving on to how and why EFT Tapping works is "pattern interrupt." A pattern interrupt is an NLP, neuro-linguistic programming, term. It is anything that creates an abrupt change.

You are having a conversation with a friend. Mid-sentence, they stop talking, reach out and put their hand on your arm. You are startled when the conversation comes to an abrupt end. Even more surprised when they put their hand on your arm. Pattern interrupt.

Part of the effectiveness of tapping is the "pattern interrupt" of energy flowing along the meridians. Dysfunctional beliefs, painful memories, and past traumas can block energy from flowing freely. Tapping on various energy points can release stagnant and blocked energy. When energy is able to flow

freely, health is restored. When healthy, the body will auto-matically gravitate to well-being, prosperity, and happiness.
In a confused state, it is difficult to know our Truths, the nitty-gritty of ourselves. By tapping, we become more of who we are and who we are meant to be as the blocks are released.

This might be a good time to also discuss tapping on one side or both sides simultaneously. In traditional Chinese medicine, there are twelve major meridians that run on each side of the body, one side mirroring the other.

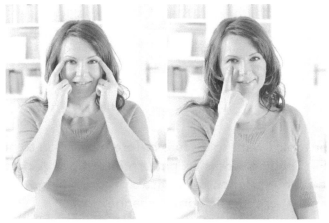

Most Effective

When the Discovery Evening group tapped both sides simul-taneously, most found statements were not clearing. How-ever, when they only tapped one side at a time, statements were clearing and there were a lot of yawns. The group and I concluded that tapping one side was more effective than tap-ping both sides. Tapping both sides was not as much of a pat-tern interrupt since the meridians flow on both sides. Tap-ping one side was more of a pattern interrupt.

Chapter 8
How Does EFT Tapping Work?

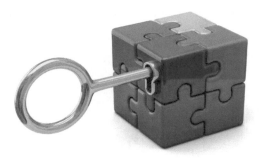

Having an understanding of an EFT Tapping statement and a pattern interrupt might help you comprehend how EFT Tapping actually works.

1. ACCEPTANCE: The last part of the tapping statement, we say, "I totally and completely accept myself." Acceptance brings us into present time. We can only heal if we are in present time.

2. ADDRESSES THE CURRENT DYSFUNCTIONAL BELIEFS ON A SUB-CONSCIOUS LEVEL: To make changes in our lives, we have to eliminate dysfunctional beliefs on a subconscious level. The middle part of the tapping statements are the "instructions" for the subconscious.

3. PATTERN INTERRUPT: Dysfunctional memories and/or beliefs block energy from flowing freely along traditional Chinese meridians. Tapping is a pattern interrupt that disrupts the flow of energy to allow our body's own Infinite Wisdom to come forth for healing. For the EFT Tapping statement "I fear change" and the client does fear change:

* This statement agrees with the current dysfunctional belief and, thus appeases the physical body. We won't be distracted as we tap.

* The tapping disrupts the energy flow so our Truth can come forth.

Chapter 9
Benefits of EFT Tapping

EFT Tapping is an evidence-based self-help tool to improve our physical, mental, and emotional well-being. There are over one hundred studies conducted in ten different countries by more than sixty researchers demonstrating EFT Tapping's effectiveness and success.

It can help reduce anxiety, stress, and food cravings. It has proven helpful for those enduring PTSD, depression, addictions, and chronic pain. Tapping can increase energy levels and reduce fatigue. Research has found that it significantly increases athletic performance. It can reduce muscular tension and joint pain. Sleeping better and less pain resulted in greater happiness and joy!

EFT Tapping can change:

Beliefs

Emotions

Self-images

Our story

Thoughts

Mind chatter

Painful memories

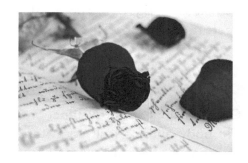

HERE ARE TEN BENEFITS OF EFT TAPPING:

1. Eliminate Dysfunctional Beliefs and Emotions
To transform our lives, we need to delete and/or modify our beliefs on a subconscious level. EFT Tapping has the potential to change our lives by eliminating the unhealthy beliefs and emotions on a subconscious level.

The natural state for the body is health and well-being. Blocked energy causes dis-ease. When we cut our finger, our body knows how to heal the cut itself. Once dysfunctional emotions, experiences, and beliefs have been "deleted," our body automatically gravitates to health, wealth, peace, love, and joy.

2. Reduce Stress and Anxiety
Research has shown that tapping can significantly decrease cortisol (stress hormone) levels and quiet the amygdala (stress center in the brain). This helps us to feel calmer and think more clearly. Less stress led to improved sleep which re-sulted in feeling more energized and less fatigued. The resting 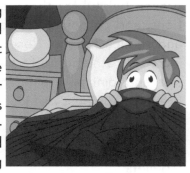 heart rate and blood pressure were reduced as well.

3. Changes Are Permanent
Once an unhealthy, dysfunctional belief has been eliminated, the body automatically gravitates to well-being. As a result, the changes we make with EFT are permanent.

4. Diminish Food Cravings and Increase Weight Loss

A study of ninety-six overweight adults was conducted in 2018. After four weeks of tapping, brain scans showed changes in the part of the brain associated with cravings. The participants reported less interest in food. Tapping can help with weight loss by creating changes in parts of the brain that activate food cravings.

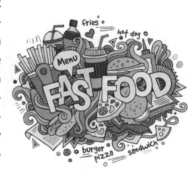

Overeating and emotional eating are symptoms of unresolved issues underneath the desire to eat. Not only has tapping been found to help cope with the physical urge to binge and emotionally eat, but it has also helped to heal the core issues around the need to overeat.

5. Improved Emotional Well-being
By eliminating the unhealthy beliefs that result in anger, fear, and/or sadness, we feel happier, our attitudes improve, and we are more optimistic about life.

6. Post Traumatic Stress Disorder (PTSD) and Other Traumas

PTSD is not limited to war veterans. Involvement in any sort of accident, surviving a natural disaster, school shootings, being told one has a terminal disease, victims of assault including sexual assault, all of these can leave one traumatized and suffering from PTSD.

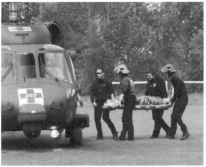 PTSD has been the subject of many studies. Research studies have found that EFT Tapping significantly decreased and/or resolved participants' PTSD, reducing flashbacks and nightmares, insomnia, trouble concentrating, isolation, hypervigilance, and aggression.

In a 2013 study, 60% of war vets felt their PTSD had been resolved after three tapping sessions. Another 30% felt their PTSD had been resolved after six tapping sessions.

7. Desensitize Emotions
We might have a difficult person in our life that ignores and/or criticizes us, so we tap the statement: "This difficult person [or their name] ignores and criticizes me."

Tapping does not mean they will no longer ignore and/or criticize us; however, it can desensitize us, so we are no longer affected by their behavior. Once we have desensitized the emotions, our perception and mental thinking improves. We are better able to make informed decisions. We don't take and make everything personal. Our health is not negatively impacted. Our hearts no longer beat 100 beats/minute, smoke stops coming out of our ears, and our faces don't turn red with anger and frustration anymore.

8. Reduce Pain and Headaches
Numerous research studies have found that EFT Tapping has helped to reduce the frequency and severity of headaches as well as reduce chronic pain.

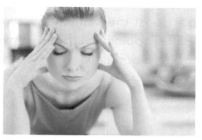

One study of people suffering from frequent tension-type headaches found that routine tapping twice a day for two months reduced both the frequency and intensity of tension headaches.

In another study of people with fibromyalgia, participants found that after an eight-week tapping program, their levels of pain were reduced.

Another study focused on people who had just undergone surgery. Five minutes of tapping for three days post-surgery significantly decreased pain levels compared to those who received no tapping treatment.

9. Athletic Performance
Various research studies have found that EFT Tapping has improved athletic per-formance. One study with female and male basketball players showed im-proved performance after fifteen min-utes of EFT Tapping compared to players who did not tap. Another study with soc-cer players showed significant improve-

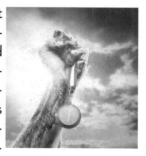

ment in goal scoring as a result of tapping. With other ath-letes, EFT Tapping helped their mental mindset, increased self-confidence, and reduced performance anxiety.

10. Boost the Immune System
EFT Tapping has been shown to increase the production of white blood cells which can supercharge our immune system.

As an EFT Practitioner, I have used EFT Tapping to help clients experience all of the benefits listed here and have witnessed the remarkable improvement in their lives. My clients have benefited from tapping for issues that include weight loss, emotional eating, athletic performance, chronic pain, and PTSD as well as personal empowerment issues.

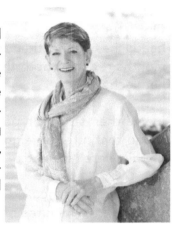

Chapter 10
The Very First EFT Tapping
Statement to Tap

The very first EFT Tapping statement I have clients and students tap is, "It is not okay or safe for my life to change." At the first session with a client, I muscle-test (a technique to ask the body questions bypassing the conscious mind), if it is okay and safe for their lives to change. No one person tested strong, that it was okay or safe for their lives to change.

I have muscle-tested this statement with more than a thousand people. Not one person tested strong that it was okay or safe for their life to change.

How effective can EFT or any therapy be
if it is not okay or safe for our lives to change?

Since our lives are constantly changing, if it is not okay or safe for our lives to change, it creates stress for the body every time it does. Stress creates another whole set of issues for ourselves, our lives, and our bodies.

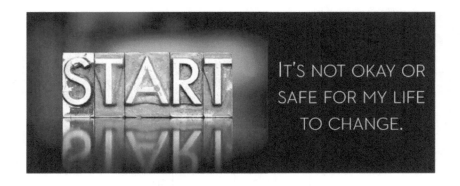

IT'S NOT OKAY OR
SAFE FOR MY LIFE
TO CHANGE.

Chapter 11
Yawning and Taking a Deep Breath

From traditional Chinese Medicine, we know that when chi (energy) flows freely through the meridians, the body is healthy and balanced. When the energy is blocked, it can result in physical, mental, and/or emotional illness.

Dysfunctional beliefs and emotions block energy from flowing freely in the body.

With EFT Tapping, as we tap, we release the blocks. As blocked energy is able to flow more freely, the body can now "breathe a sigh of relief." Yawning is that sigh of relief.

If, after tapping, we can take a complete, deep, full, and satisfying breath, we know that an EFT Tapping statement has cleared.

If the yawn or breath is not a full, deep breath then the statement did not clear completely.

Chapter 12
Integration...What Happens
After Tapping

After tapping, our system needs some downtime for integration to take place. When the physical body and the mind are "idle," integration can take place.

Sometimes, in the first 24 hours after tapping, we might find ourselves sleeping more than normal or feeling more tired. This downtime is needed to integrate the new changes.

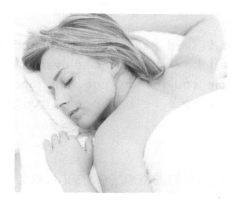

After installing a new program on our computer, sometimes we have to reboot the computer (shut down and restart) for the new program to be integrated into the system.

After tapping, our bodies need to reboot. We need some downtime. When we sleep, the new changes are integrated.

HEALING BEGINS NATURALLY AFTER THE BODY
HAS HAD A CHANCE TO INTEGRATE.

Sometimes, after tapping, we forget the intensity of our pain and think that feeling better has nothing to do with tapping. Something so simple could not possibly be the reason for the improvement!

When we cut our finger, once it is healed, we don't remember cutting our finger. As we move toward health, wealth, and well-being, sometimes we don't remember how unhappy, restless, or isolated we once felt.

I had a client, Sam. He had been struggling with an issue for twenty years. After the session, I called Sam to make sure he was okay. He said, "I'm doing great. I don't know why I needed to see you because I am all good now."

A little confused, I asked if something had happened or what he felt had caused the change to make everything great now. He said, "No." He couldn't imagine that tapping his head would change an issue he had been struggling with for twenty years!

Tapping is a simple exercise that has long-lasting,
meaningful results for a tapper

Chapter 13
Intensity Level

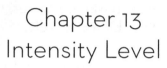

One measure of knowing how much an issue has improved is by giving the issue an intensity number (IL) between 1 and 10, 1 being low and with 10 being high. This is done before tapping begins and reassessed throughout the tapping process.

For example, we want a romantic partnership, yet we haven't met "the one." Thinking about a romantic relationship happening, what is the likelihood, on a scale of 1 – 10, with 10 being very likely and 1, not likely at all, of a romantic relationship happening.

After thinking about it, and checking with our inner self, we give ourselves a 2 for the likelihood of a romantic relationship happening. Now, let's start tapping.

When asked what the issues might be, "Well," we say, "It does not seem as if the people I want, want me."

Great tapping statement. Tap, "Even though the people I want don't want me, I totally and completely accept myself." After tapping, we check in with ourselves; the IL has gone up to a 4, so it is now a little bit more likely.

What comes to mind now? "No one will find me desirable." Great tapping statement. "Even though no one will find me desirable, I totally and completely accept myself." Check the IL. How likely? 5. Cool! Progress.

What comes to mind now? "I'm not comfortable being vulnerable in romantic relationships." Great tapping statement. "Even though I'm not comfortable being vulnerable in a romantic relationship, I totally and completely accept myself." Check the IL. Now it is a 6. Still progress.

What comes to mind now? "Well, it feels like if I am in a relationship, I will lose a lot of my freedom." Make this into a tapping statement. "Even though I will lose my freedom when I am in a relationship, I totally and completely accept myself." The IL has gone up to a 7.

What comes to mind now? "Oh, if I was in a relationship, I would have to be accountable to someone!" Make this into a tapping statement: "Even though, I would have to be accountable to someone if I was in a relationship, I totally and completely accept myself." Wow...the IL is 9, very likely!

Chapter 14
Walking Backwards EFT (Backing Up)

As I was working with a client, Joanne, an issue was not clearing. Knowing that movement helps to resolve problems, I told Joanne to stand up. Joanne and I backed up, walking backward, as we spoke the tapping statements. Literally, we walked backwards, step after step, facing forward while our feet stepped backward.

Surprise, surprise, it worked. Every Statement cleared as Joanne backed up.

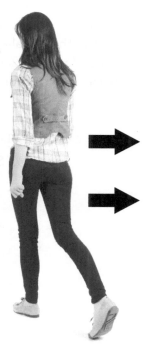

Walking forward represents forward movement in our lives. Walking backward represents the past.

Physical movement can help clear emotional issues and facilitate change.

Walking backward undoes the past and helps to clear, heal, and transform an issue in our lives.

The next client, Bill, came in for his session. I had him walk backwards. His issues were being resolved as well by backing up. Both Joanne and Bill are somewhat athletic and workout. I wanted to know if the backing up would work with non-athletic people. I was teaching an EFT class that night. At the end of the class, we all backed up together. And, IT WORKED!

Let's say we want to process, "I will never be comfortable in the world." Stand up. Make sure nothing is behind you. Then walk backward while facing forward and say, "I will never be comfortable in the world. I will never be comfortable in the world. I will never be comfortable in the world. I will never be comfortable in the world." Repeat the phrase six to eight times.

Initially, as Bill and Joanne began walking backwards, it was difficult for them to keep their balance. As the statement cleared, their balance and ability to walk backwards improved. Joanne exclaimed, "I can tell when the statement begins to clear because I stand taller and my balance improves."

Backing up EFT worked with every client and student. How cool is that!

Chapter 15
Two Styles of Tapping

Laser-focused Tapping vs Round Robin Tapping

The Discovery Evening group and I explored different issues, situations, and memories to determine how best to resolve and heal different issues in our lives.

With Johnnie not feeling good enough, his situation was more about the beliefs he had about himself. Beliefs such as:

* I will always be rejected because I am not good enough.
* I have to be perfect so others won't see my flaws.
* It's not safe to show others the real me.
* I will never succeed in life.

Kala's situation was different. She had been dating a man for two years and thought he was "the one." She and Steve had talked about marriage, buying a home together, and having a family. They knew each other's likes and dislikes, how they each felt about disciplining children, and what each other's life-long goals were. Kala began reading wedding magazines, and visualizing her wedding gown, and the ceremony.

Three days passed and she had not heard from Steve. She decided to stop by his home. Out front was a "For Rent" sign! A few days later, she received an email from Steve.

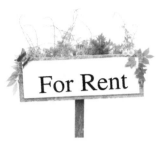

Steve's work offered him a promotion outside the country. He wasn't sure what he wanted to do and didn't want anyone pressuring him to make a decision. He needed to determine what was best for him. Ultimately, he took the new position and ended the relationship with Kala.

Two different situations, each benefitted from a different style of tapping. What the group and I concluded was that "laser-focused tapping," making the same statement for all eight points was best for healing dysfunctional beliefs. The beliefs Johnnie had about "not being good enough" would benefit from this style of tapping.

Round robin tapping, scripts, was best for healing emotions, desensitizing a story, situation, and/or memory. Kala would benefit from the round robin/script tapping to desensitize her crushed heart.

Laser Focused Tapping
Same Statement for all the Tapping Points in One Round

Example: After tapping the statement, "It's not okay for my life to change," if we are able to take a deep breath, we know the statement has cleared. Then if we tap, "I'm not ready for my life to change," and we are not able to take a deep breath, most likely, the statement did not clear.

Circling under the collar bone:

1. Even though, it is not ready for my life to change, I totally and completely accept myself.

2. Even though, it is not ready for my life to change, I totally and completely accept myself.

3. Even though, it is not ready for my life to change, I totally and completely accept myself.

Tapping:

Eyebrow – It's not ready for my life to change.
Temple – It's not ready for my life to change.
Side of the eye - It's not ready for my life to change.
Under the eye – It's not ready for my life to change.
Under the nose – It's not ready for my life to change.
Under the lips – It's not ready for my life to change.
Collar bone knob – It's not ready for my life to change.
Top back of head – It's not ready for my life to change.

Knowing the statement did not clear, we can focus on the reasons, excuses, and/or beliefs about not being ready to change our lives.

* Maybe the changes we need to make would require more of us than we want to give.
* Maybe we don't feel we have the abilities we would need if our life changed.
* Maybe we don't feel our support system, the people in our life, would approve of the changes we want to make.

Follow-up tapping statements for "I'm not ready for my life to change" could be:

* I do not have the abilities change would require.
* I am afraid of change.
* Others will not support the changes I want to make in my life.
* I am not able to make the changes I want to make.
* I do not have the courage that change would require.
* I am too old to change.

Tapping the same statement at all eight points is most effective for clearing beliefs. When a statement does not clear, we can then focus on the reasons, excuses, and/or dysfunctional beliefs that blocked the statement from clearing.

SCRIPTS/ROUND ROBIN
MULTIPLE STATEMENTS IN ONE ROUND OF TAPPING

Tapping multiple statements in one round, also known as Scripts or Round Robin tapping, is excellent for healing a story or desensitizing a memory.

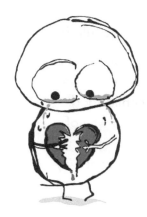

To desensitize the heartache of the break up, the following script/statements could be said, one statement per tapping point:

Eyebrow – My boyfriend broke up with me.

Temple – I am heartbroken.

Side of the eye - He said he doesn't love me anymore.

Under the eye – I don't know how I can go on without him.

Under the nose – It hurts.

Under the lips – I am sad he doesn't love me anymore.

Collar bone knob – I am sad our relationship is over.

Top back of head – I will never find anyone like him ever again.

Reframing

Reframing is a Neuro-Linguistic Programming (NLP) term. It is a way to view and experience emotions, situations, and/or behaviors in a more positive manner.

At the end of round robin tapping, we can introduce statements to "reframe" the situation.

An example of reframing could be:

* I want to eat this chocolate cake.
* Maybe eating chocolate is a way to reconnect to my childhood.
* Maybe eating sugar is a way of being loved.
* Maybe I can find a different way of being loved.

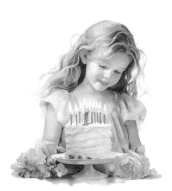

Round robin tapping, scripts, can desensitize the hurt and pain. It can heal the pain of our story. It may not rewrite the beliefs. To clear the beliefs, it would be necessary to look at the reasons the relationship didn't work and why our heart is broken or why we crave chocolate.

Round robin/script tapping can also be done by just tapping the side of the hand.

SIDE OF HAND (SOH) TAPPING TO DESENSITIZE A STORY, SITUATION, AND/OR MEMORY

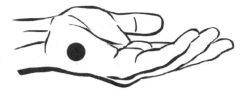

When our lives have been turned upside down and inside out because of something that happened, it is best to neutralize the event. If a memory still haunts us, we can tap the side of the hand as we reflect on the event.

As Sasha, another client of mine, was telling her story, tears filled her eyes. I had her tap the side of her hand as she recalled her worst high school dance ever!

As Sasha tapped the side of the hand, she said: My best friend, Samantha and I, were so excited about attending our first high school dance. We weren't old enough to drive so Sam's dad dropped us off in front of the high school auditorium where the dance was held.

(Continuing to tap the SOH) We were in awe of how the auditorium was transformed into a palace. Sofas were placed around a hardwood dance floor in the center of the room. We promised to be there for each other throughout the night so neither of us would be stranded alone.

(Continuing to tap the SOH) Well, along came Billy McDaniels. Sam had had a crush on Billy since third grade. He asked her to dance. I never saw her again for the rest of the night.

(Continuing to tap the SOH) Those three hours were proba-bly the worst night of my entire life! No one asked me to dance. Every time I joined a group of girls, a new song would begin, and every one of them was asked to dance, everyone except me. I don't know why no one asked me to dance. I felt ugly, abandoned, and undesirable! Talk about being a wall-flower. I thought I was invisible. I wanted to hide from embar-rassment.

(Continuing to tap the SOH) This was back in the days before cell phones. The auditorium didn't have a payphone to call my parents to come and get me. I had to endure three hours of humiliation, watching every single girl be asked to dance EX-CEPT me.

(Continuing to tap the SOH) I never attended another high school dance again!

Whether we tap the side of our hand or the eight tapping points, the result is the same. Round robin tapping can de-sensitize emotions and memories very effectively.

There are different styles of EFT Tapping.
Find the style that works best for your desired result.

Chapter 16
EFT Tapping Doesn't Work for Me

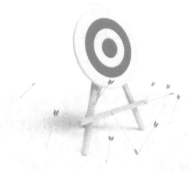

EFT Tapping works best when

1) the statements are worded to eliminate dysfunctional beliefs,
2) the most effective style of tapping is utilized, and
3) we are healing the cause, not just the symptoms.

If an issue doesn't seem to be resolved after tapping, ask yourself the following questions:

* Were the statements worded so that a dysfunctional belief and/or emotion could be addressed and eliminated?

* Was the best style of tapping (laser-focused vs scripts) utilized?

* Were the tapping statements addressing the symptom or the cause?

For EFT Tapping to be effective,
the cause of the issue needs to be healed.

* Having an awareness of our issues does not heal dysfunctional beliefs.
* Forgiving ourselves and/or someone else does not heal dysfunctional beliefs.
* Talk therapy does not heal dysfunctional beliefs.
* Desensitizing emotions does not heal dysfunctional beliefs.
* Healing the experience of a hurtful event does not change dysfunctional beliefs.

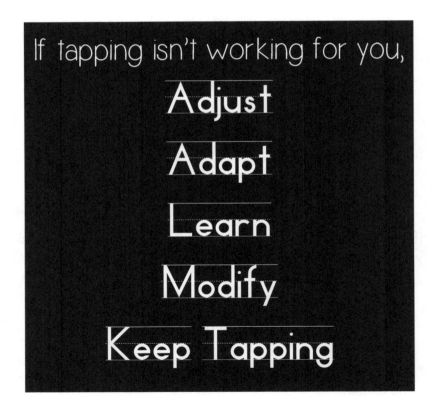

If tapping isn't working for you,

Adjust

Adapt

Learn

Modify

Keep Tapping

Chapter 17
What to Do If an EFT Tapping Statement Does Not Clear

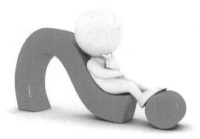

When a statement might not clear, turn the statement into a question. If the statement, "It's not okay for me to be powerful," didn't clear, **turn the tapping statement into a question:** "Why isn't it okay for me to be powerful?"

The answer might be:

* Powerful people are ruthless and heartless.
* I am afraid of being powerful.
* Being powerful would change me for the worse.
* Power corrupts.
* People would laugh at me if I tried being powerful.
* I might be called aggressive if I tried being powerful.
* I don't have the abilities, skills, or qualities to be powerful.
* Powerful people are thoughtless and self-centered.

With these beliefs, it might not be okay or safe to be powerful or even explore the idea of being powerful. The statements above are tapping statements. Tap the answer to the question.

After tapping the answer(s) to the question, revisit the original statement that did not clear. Most likely, it will now be cleared, and you will be able to take a full, deep, and complete breath.

If not, ask more questions and tap the answers. What we tapped, cleared. If you are not able to take a deep breath after tapping, the bottom-line cause has not been found yet. Keep asking questions and tapping until the underlying cause has been discovered and healed.

DO I KEEP TAPPING THE SAME STATEMENT IF IT DOESN'T CLEAR?

Tapping round after round after round, repeating the same statement over and over again as we tap does not ensure success.

For example: we tapped, "It is not okay or safe for me to be wealthy." It did not clear after one round of EFT Tapping. We truly want to be wealthy, so we continue to tap, round after round and the statement will not clear. We must dig deeper into other beliefs we have.

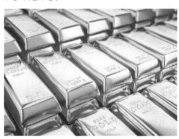

What other beliefs might we have about money?

* It is not okay for me to have more than others.
* People might try to manipulate me for my money.
* My spending might get out of control.
* Others would think I am arrogant and better than them if I
  had money.

With beliefs such as these, it might not be okay or safe to be wealthy. Rather than tapping round after round after round of the same statement, turn the statement into a question and tap the answers. "Well, why would it not be okay or safe for me to be wealthy?"

The answer you might discover is:

* I do not have the tools and skills to manage money.
* I have to work hard for my money.
* It is too much stress to maintain a wealthy lifestyle.
* The economy is too volatile and unpredictable. I might end
  up losing my wealth.

Once you uncover the additional beliefs and tap those statements, the previous statement(s) that did not clear most likely will have cleared.

An Issue Keeps Showing Up in My Life After Tapping

"I processed the issue I had, and I am not any better. Why?"

When we tap and process an issue, and the issue persists, it is not the process that did not work; it is the issue we processed. The correct CAUSE was not processed.

For instance, we resist change and often say, "I know I need to change, but..."

* Is the issue our resistance to change, or do we lack something to move toward?

* We process being stuck in the past, but the real issue might be that we have nothing to move forward to in the future.

* Maybe it is about our lack of goals or not having the skills to fulfill a goal.

* Maybe it is our lack of dreams and believing this is the best our life will ever be.

For instance, we may feel it is selfish to put ourselves and our needs first.

* Something bad will happen to those we love if we do not put them first.

* Others might call me selfish if I take care of my needs before theirs.

So, we process our selfishness. We process what others might say or think if we put ourselves first. Maybe the issue is not what others will think and say. Maybe the issue is us. Maybe we are just not that important to ourselves. Maybe the issue is self-love, self-respect, and self-worth.

When we process, and the same issue persists,
it is not the process that did not work.
It is the issue we processed

For example, our eating is out of control. So, we process this issue, but our eating remains out of control. Maybe the issue is not about our eating being out of control.

* Maybe the issue is about stress or lack of self-confidence or anger, fear, and/or apathy that result in overeating.

* Maybe the issue is the lack of control we feel we have in our life.

* Maybe our out-of-control eating is a symptom that our life is out of balance.

If we process and the issue seems to persist, look at the issue again, but from a different perspective. Flip it around. Look at it from the opposite perspective.

Process this new perspective.

* It might be about the future, not the past.

* It might be about our self-respect rather than someone else's respect for us.

* Maybe it is a symptom of another issue.

Flip it around
Look at the issue from another perspective

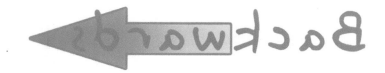

Chapter 18
Does a Negative Statement Parrot My Negative Self-Talk?

A tapping statement with the word "no" or "not" may sound like our inner critic and/or our negative self-talk. Our inner critic and negative self-talk are actually our teachers. They are letting us know the dysfunctional beliefs we need to change to advance toward health, wealth, and well-being.

Since we ignore their words of wisdom, it seems as if our inner voice is critical and negative, as if they are nagging us. The truth is this: They are pointing out what needs to be healed in order for us to be healthy, wealthy, happy, and wise!

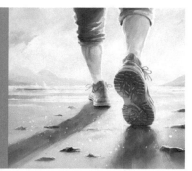

Our inner critic and
negative self-talk
are words of pearls
shining a light
on the path that
needs to be healed

For example, let's say our negative self-talk goes something like this, "I will never lose the weight." What might the body be trying to tell us?

* Maybe the beliefs of being able to lose weight need to be examined and healed.

* Maybe it is about being visible and present or dealing with the anger and shame beneath the weight or about our fear of intimacy and closeness.

The body has an Infinite Wisdom. It will always gravitate toward health, peace, and joy. When we tap, we are calling forth our Truths, our Infinite Wisdom. EFT Tapping will not change our Truth. Gravity exists on Earth. Tapping will not change whether I would be affected by gravity or not.

We cannot gravitate to health, peace, wealth, and joy if we are being prevented from doing so. "Blocked energy," or energy that is not able to flow freely in the body, prevents us from gravitating to wellness, prosperity, and happiness.

Energy that is able to flow freely
will allow our bodies to heal

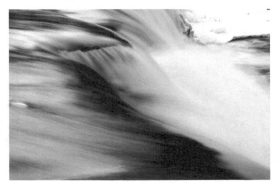

Chapter 19
Science and EFT Tapping Research

EFT has been researched in more than ten countries by over sixty investigators whose results have been published in more than twenty different peer-reviewed journals. Two leading researchers are Dawson Church, Ph.D. and David Feinstein, Ph.D.

Dr. Dawson Church, a leading expert on energy psychology and an EFT master, has gathered all the research information, and it can be found on this website: www.EFTUniverse.com.

TWO RESEARCH STUDIES

1) HARVARD MEDICAL SCHOOL STUDIES AND THE BRAIN'S STRESS RESPONSE

Studies at the Harvard Medical School reveal that tapping points along energy meridians significantly reduces activity in a part of the brain called the amygdala.

The amygdala can be thought of as the body's alarm system. When the body is experiencing trauma or fear, the amygdala is triggered, and the body is flooded with cortisol, also known as the stress hormone.

2) DR. DAWSON CHURCH AND CORTISOL REDUCTION

Another significant study was conducted by Dr. Dawson Church. He studied the impact an hour's tapping session had on the cortisol levels of eighty-three subjects. He also measured the cortisol levels of people who received traditional talk therapy and those of a third group who received no treatment at all.

On average, for the eighty-three subjects who completed an hour tapping session, cortisol levels were reduced by 24%. Some subjects experienced a 50% reduction in cortisol levels.

The subjects who completed one hour of traditional talk therapy and those who received neither therapies (tapping or talk therapy), did not experience any significant cortisol reduction.

With hundreds of research studies, EFT Tapping is an evidence-based self-help tool that has been proven to improve our physical, mental, and emotional well-being.

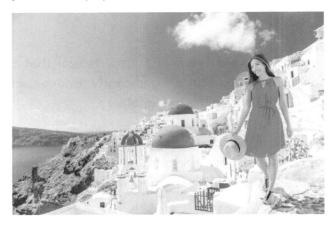

Chapter 20
Is Lowering Our Cortisol Levels Enough to Change Our Lives Permanently?

Several things can lower our cortisol (stress hormone) levels, including:

* Power posing (superman and wonder woman pose with hands on waist)
* Meditating
* Laughing
* Exercising regularly
* Listening to music
* Getting a massage
* Eliminating caffeine from our diet
* Eating a balanced, nutritious meal and eliminating processed food

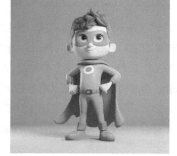

Would performing any of the above activities lower our cortisol levels enough to permanently change our lives? Only if the activity eliminates dysfunctional beliefs on a subconscious level.

All of our thoughts, feelings, actions, reactions, choices, and decisions are preceded by a belief. To change our lives, dysfunctional beliefs must be eliminated.

Power posing, listening to music, or eating a balanced meal will not permanently change our lives. Exercising will help our physical body but will not delete our dysfunctional beliefs. Laughing will bring us into the present so we will not be drawn into our fears or anger, but it will not change our lives. Meditating helps us to center and balance, but it will not change our lives on a permanent basis.

To change our lives, we must recognize, acknowledge, and take ownership of what we want to change, and then delete dysfunctional emotions and beliefs on the subconscious level.

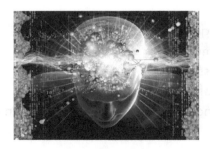

EFT Tapping will delete dysfunctional emotions and beliefs on a subconscious level if we provide the correct "instructions" to our subconscious mind. We must word the tapping statements in the subconscious' language. We must word the tapping statement so the subconscious mind hears what we want to eliminate.

Chapter 21
Tapping Affirmations

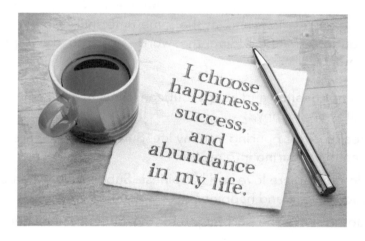

Do you repeat these affirmations?

1. I am healthy and happy.
2. Wealth is pouring into my life.
3. I radiate love and happiness.
4. I have the perfect job for me.
5. I am successful in whatever I do.

If we were to tap "I am healthy and happy now" and we are not, most likely, as we are tapping, we might think, "Yeah, right. Sure. I am healthy and happy. My life sucks. I hate my job. I am always broke. There is never enough money."

The body knows this is not true. We are not healthy and happy now. When we tap, we might have difficulty remembering what we are saying, lose focus and concentration, and/or the mind drifts.

An EFT Tapping statement is most
effective **when** it matches our current belief.

The subconscious does not hear the word "No." One way of tapping affirmations and, at the same time, increase our positive outlook, is by adding the word "no" into the tapping statements.

1. I am **not** healthy and happy. Subconscious hears: I am healthy and happy.
2. Wealth is **not** pouring into my life. Subconscious hears: Wealth is pouring into my life.
3. I **do not** radiate love and happiness. Subconscious hears: I radiate love and happiness.
4. I **do not** have the perfect job for me. Subconscious hears: I have the perfect job for me.
5. I am **not** successful in whatever I do. Subconscious hears: I am successful in whatever I do.

If we repeat affirmations over and over before we clear the affirmation with EFT Tapping, it will have little effect. Repeating affirmations creates circumstances in our lives where we are confronted by our beliefs that do not align with the affirmation.

For affirmations to be most beneficial, tap the
affirmation by adding a "no" to the tapping statement.

Chapter 22
Finishing Touches –
Positive Statements

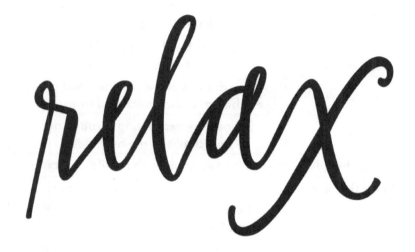

Some people like to finish their tapping with statements that are centering and calming. If this is you, then you might want to try the sixteen statements on the next page or make up those that you like. The statements can be said in any order that works for you.

Tapping Location	Statement
Eyebrow	All is well in my life.
Temple	Every day in every way I am getting better and better.
Under the Eye	I am fulfilled in every way, every day.
Under the Nose	My blessings appears in rich appropriate form with divine timing.
Under the Lips	I am an excellent steward of wealth and am blessed with great abundance.
Under the Collar- bone Knob	I take complete responsibility for everything in my life.
Under the Arm	I have all the tools, skills, and abilities to excel in my life.
Top back part of the Head	I know I will be able to handle anything that arises in my life.
Eyebrow	All my dreams, hopes, wishes, and goals are being fulfilled each and every day.
Temple	Divine love expressing through me, now draws to me new ideas.
Under the Eye	I am comfortable with my life changing.
Under the Nose	I am able to create all that I desire.
Under the Lips	I know what needs to be done and follow through to completion.
Under the Collar- bone Knob	My health is perfect in every way, physically, mentally, emotionally, and spiritually.
Under the Arm	I invite into my subconscious Archangel Raphael to heal all that needs to be forgiven, released, and redeemed. Cleanse me and free me from it now.
Top back part of the Head	The light of God surrounds me. The love of God enfolds me. The power of God protects me. The presence of God watches over and flows through me.

Chapter 23 – How to Use This Book

1. The statements are divided into sections. Read through the statements in one section. Notice if you have any reaction to the statement or feel the statement might be true for you. If so, note the number for that statement.

2. List the top seven or more statements.

3. From this list, select one and describe how it plays out in your life. It is important to recognize and identify the patterns, the consequences of having this belief, the trigger(s), and how it begins.

4. Tap the statements. Statements can be combined for scripts.

5. After tapping, review the statements to determine if you still have a reaction to any of the statements or you do not think the statement cleared. If you do, you have several options:
A) Put a "Why" before the statement. Tap the answers.
B) Keep a list of statements that do not clear. After additional tapping, return to this list to determine if the statement has cleared. Statements that still have not cleared, put a "why" before the statement and tap the answers.

6. Allow some downtime for integration and the body to heal.

7. The number of sections you do at a time will be up to you. Initially, you might want to do one section to determine if you get tired and need to have some downtime after tapping.

Chapter 24
EFT Tapping Statements 1 – 20

*Worrying is like a rocking chair. It gives you
something to do, but it gets you nowhere.*

Glenn Turner

1. I never do enough.
2. I worry all the time.
3. I can't stop worrying.
4. I will fail if I take a risk.
5. I am my harshest critic.
6. I stew about my future.
7. I avoid being in a crowd.
8. I worry about everything.
9. I am my own worst enemy.
10. I cringe when I am criticized.
11. I check and recheck my work.
12. I numb out when I am anxious.
13. I magnify my faults and errors.
14. Worry is a natural state for me.
15. I have a lot of trouble relaxing.
16. I must do everything correctly.
17. It is not okay/safe to take risks.
18. I go over and over the "what ifs."
19. I am uncomfortable with change.
20. I will never get over my anxieties.

Journaling for Statements 1 - 20

Your biggest problem or difficulty today has been sent to you at this moment to teach you something you need to know to be happier and more successful in the future.

Brian Tracy

1. From the tapping statements between 1 - 20, tap the top seven statements that you thought or felt applied to you:

1.

2.

3.

4.

5.

6.

7.

2. From this list above, select one and describe how it plays out in your life. Give an example. It is important to recognize and identify the pattern, triggers, how it begins, how has it benefited and harmed you? For instance, you lack direction, purpose, and meaning in your life and don't have a clue what your life is about. Is it easier to worry than to define your life, find meaning in life?

EFT Tapping Statements 21 – 40

*You can't wring your hands and roll
up your sleeves at the same time.*

Pat Schroeder

21. I cannot tolerate being out of control.

22. I couldn't stop worrying even if I tried.

23. I know my panic attacks will never end.

24. I find it difficult to take life as it comes.

25. I go into overwhelm when I am anxious.

26. I am highly critical of my performances.

27. I have to be the best at everything I do.

28. I don't have any control of my thoughts.

29. I stuff and suppress my anxious feelings.

30. I am anxious when I begin a new activity.

31. I have difficulty controlling my worrying.

32. My favorite saying seems to be "if only."

33. My favorite saying seems to be "what if."

34. It is not safe for me to ignore my worries.

35. The more inferior I feel, the more I worry.

36. I am defined by my anxieties and worries.

37. I blame others when I am feeling anxious.

38. My mind worries whether I want to or not.

39. I cannot handle scary situations or people.

40. My worry keeps me keyed up and restless.

Journaling for Statements 21 – 40

If you see ten troubles coming down the road, you can be sure that nine will run into the ditch before they reach you

Calvin Coolidge

1. From the tapping statements between 21 – 40, tap the top seven statements that you thought or felt applied to you:

1.

2.

3.

4.

5.

6.

7.

2. From this list above, select one and describe how it plays out in your life. Give an example. It is important to recognize and identify the pattern, triggers, how it begins, how has it benefited and harmed you? For instance, do you stew about your future? The future happens in the present. We take action in the present for what we want to create in the future. What are you doing to create your future now? Do you know what you want in the future? Are you willing to do the work to make your future a reality?

EFT Tapping Statements 41 – 60

Worry never robs tomorrow of its
sorrow. It only saps today of its joy.

Leo Buscaglia

41. The worse always happens to me.
42. I make mountains out of molehills.
43. I am not comfortable in the world.
44. My anxiety haunts me all day long.
45. My worrying does serve a purpose.
46. Worrying demonstrates that I care.
47. I don't know how to manage stress.
48. I can't cope with difficult situations.
49. I should not/cannot make mistakes.
50. I don't know how to solve problems.
51. I focus on the worse-case scenarios.
52. I am anxious about most everything.
53. The world is a very dangerous place.
54. It is difficult for me to stop worrying.
55. I turn errors into major catastrophes.
56. I avoid traveling away from my home.
57. I will never be able to let my fears go.
58. I am overly sensitive to others' needs.
59. I am apprehensive when I am anxious.
60. I lack social skills to be around others.

Journaling for Statements 41 – 60

You can't make footprints in the sand of time if you're sitting on your butt and who wants to make butt prints in the sand of time?

Bob Moawad

1. From the tapping statements between 41 – 60, tap the top seven statements that you thought or felt applied to you:

1.

2.

3.

4.

5.

6.

7.

2. From this list above, select one and describe how it plays out in your life. Give an example. It is important to recognize and identify the pattern, triggers, how it begins, how has it benefited and harmed you? For instance, is anxiety the primary motivating force in your life? If your life was peaceful, would you be less productive? Or do you think that others would find fault with you and think you aren't doing enough if you were calm and centered?

EFT Tapping Statements 61 – 80

*You can't wring your hands and roll
up your sleeves at the same time.*

Pat Schroeder

61. I torture myself with worse-case scenarios.
62. I handle my anxiety by being super-human.
63. It is not safe to take care of my needs first.
64. I should be able to foresee every difficulty.
65. I should be doing more than what I do now.
66. I push aside my needs for the people I love.
67. I am susceptible to the negativity of others.
68. I handle my anxiety by being a perfectionist.
69. I worry when I feel vulnerable and insecure.
70. I am constantly comparing myself to others.
71. A terrible event will happen if I don't worry.
72. My life is about pain, struggle, and suffering.
73. I worry most about _____, _____, and _____.
74. I don't trust that things will work out for me.
75. I worry without reaching a possible solution.
76. I am powerless to live my life any differently.
77. My anxiety interferes with my ability to work.
78. My thoughts get jumbled when I am anxious.
79. I handle my anxiety by being an overachiever.
80. I use "never" and "always" to describe myself.

Journaling for Statements 61 - 80

*If we actively do something, it will stop making us feel
like a victim and we'll start feeling like part of the solution,
which is a huge benefit to our body and your psyche.*

Ted Danson

1. From the tapping statements between 61 - 80, tap the top
seven statements that you thought or felt applied to you:

1.

2.

3.

4.

5.

6.

7.

2. From this list above, select one and describe how it plays
out in your life. Give an example. It is important to recognize
and identify the pattern, triggers, how it begins, how has it
benefited and harmed you? For instance, do you minimize
your strengths, abilities, talents, and achievements? Is this
about being noticed and seen? Or do you think that more
would be expected of you if you were strong, able, and tal-
ented?

EFT Tapping Statements 81 – 100

I am an old man and have known a great
many troubles. Most of them never happened.

Mark Twain

81. I will never learn to be comfortable in the world.
82. My worry keeps me irritable and sleep deprived.
83. It is not safe to say "no" to a request made of me.
84. I am powerless and a victim of my circumstances.
85. Worry prevents me from making good decisions.
86. Anxiety is the primary motivating force in my life.
87. Something bad will happen when I stop worrying.
88. I worry that everything will always turn out badly.
89. My worries wake me up in the middle of the night.
90. I am anxious when there are unexpected changes.
91. I worry that someone I love will be hurt or harmed.
92. I turn small personal flaws into major catastrophes.
93. I have difficulty accepting the ups and downs of life.
94. I worry that something bad will happen in the future.
95. I am flawed, inadequate, and unacceptable to others.
96. I use my worrying as a distraction from life and living.
97. I think of all the frightening things that could happen.
98. My worrisome thoughts recycle endlessly in my mind.
99. I let others know when I am worried about something.
100. I think about fearful situations over and over and over.

Journaling for Statements 81 – 100

Sorrow looks back
Worry looks around
Faith looks ahead

Beatrice Fallon

1. From the tapping statements between 81 – 100, tap the top seven statements that you thought or felt applied to you:

1.

2.

3.

4.

5.

6.

7.

2. From this list above, select one and describe how it plays out in your life. Give an example. It is important to recognize and identify the pattern, triggers, how it begins, how has it benefited and harmed you? For instance, are you too stuck in your ways to change or change is just too difficult? Do you have goals or just drift with whatever?

EFT Tapping Statements 101 – 120

If I had my life to live over, I would perhaps have more actual troubles and fewer imaginary ones.

Don Herold

101. I should be totally competent and self-reliant.
102. My life lacks meaning, purpose, and direction.
103. I am the only one that can solve my problems.
104. I am super-sensitive to criticism and rejection.
105. I worry about a problem so it won't get worse.
106. There is just too much information to process.
107. I focus on the negative instead of the positive.
108. My anxiety and constant worrying is incurable.
109. I am always waiting for the other shoe to drop.
110. I tend to mull things over and over in my mind.
111. I don't feel satisfied unless it is done perfectly.
112. I should not do anything to make others angry.
113. I am not willing to face or deal with my anxiety.
114. I don't trust that everything will turn out A-OK.
115. I don't have the ability to overcome my anxiety.
116. I worry when everything in my life is going well.
117. My negative self-talk is the cause of my anxiety.
118. I am inferior to others, defective, and unworthy.
119. I am most anxious about _____, _____, and _____.
120. I have to have a quick answer to every problem.

Journaling for Statements 101 – 120

*It has been said that our anxiety does
not empty tomorrow of its sorrow, but
only empties today of its strength.*

Charles Haddon Spurgeon

1. From the tapping statements between 101 – 120, tap the top seven statements that you thought or felt applied to you:

1.

2.

3.

4.

5.

6.

7.

2. From this list above, select one and describe how it plays out in your life. Give an example. It is important to recognize and identify the pattern, triggers, how it begins, how has it benefited and harmed you? For instance, is it easier to worry than admit you don't have the tools and skills to handle the situation, you don't know how to take responsibility, or how to solve the problem?

EFT Tapping Statements 121 – 140

Worry bankrupts the spirit.

Berri Clove

121. I worry about all the bad things that will happen to me.

122. My anxiety makes me feel nervous, tense, and on edge.

123. Others may not think I care if I don't worry about them.

124. I overcome my anxiety by planning for all contingencies.

125. I focus so much on the details that I miss the big picture.

126. I am very concerned and anxious about making mistakes.

127. Worry is a way of preventing bad things from happening.

128. I don't know how to handle frustration, anger, and/or loss.

129. My value comes from helping others solve their problems.

130. I don't have the ability to eliminate worry whenever I want.

131. Others know I am a worry wart so they don't tell me things.

132. I am excluded a lot because all I talk about are my anxieties.

133. I minimize my strengths, abilities, talents, and achievements.

134. I can't stop talking about something when I am anxious about it.

135. I always imagine the worst-case scenario, catastrophe, and disaster.

136. I shop, gamble, and/or watch TV to distract myself from my anxiety.

137. I turn a single negative event into a never-ending pattern of defeat.

138. I don't know how to distinguish realistic worry from unrealistic worry.

139. I have a lot of "shoulds," "musts," "oughts," "have tos," and/or "can'ts."

140. I avoid specific places, events, and/or situations because of my anxiety.

Journaling for Statements 121 – 140

Worry gives a small thing a big shadow.

Swedish proverb

1. From the tapping statements between 121 – 140, tap the top seven statements that you thought or felt applied to you:

1.

2.

3.

4.

5.

6.

7.

2. From this list above, select one and describe how it plays out in your life. Give an example. It is important to recognize and identify the pattern, triggers, how it begins, how has it benefited and harmed you? For instance, do you turn a single negative event into a never-ending pattern of defeat? How does this serve you? Well, less would be expected and asked of you. You can stay in your anxiety. You don't have to progress in your life...lots of benefits to being less than successful.

New Product Launching Fall 2023

Tessa created a new series call *Awaken, Emerge, Become* to provide a guide for a seeker to find their own insights and ah-ha wisdom. The series includes a book, card deck, journal, and Workbook and work in tandem with each other.

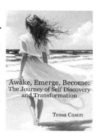

The book, *Awaken, Emerge, Become: The Journey of Self-Reflection and Transformation* is a step-by-step guide from self discovery to transformation. It includes many of the tools, techniques, and methods she learned from some remarkable teachers.

The sixty card deck, *Awaken, Emerge, Become: Card Deck of Exploration* is a fun tool to aid in finding answers, discover new insights, and might provide new awarenesses for the inquisitive.

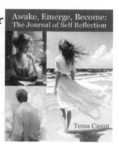

Awaken, Emerge, Become: The Journal of Self-reflection is a series of questions to help a seeker discern their truths. The intent of the journal is to assist you in finding your ah-ha wisdom, answers to the challenges you currently are facing, and possible paths to healing physically, mentally, emotionally, and spiritually.

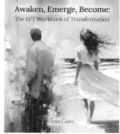

Awaken, Emerge, Become: The EFT Workbook for Transformation is a step-by-step guide to becoming the highest potential of ourselves.

Books by Tessa Cason

80 EFT TAPPING STATEMENTS FOR:
Abandonment
Abundance, Wealth, Money
Addictions
Adult Children of Alcoholics
Anger and Frustration
Anxiety and Worry
Change
"Less Than" and Anxiety
Manifesting a Romantic Relationship
Relationship with Self
Self Esteem
Social Anxiety
Weight and Emotional Eating

100 EFT Tapping Statements for Accepting Our Uniqueness
and Being Different
100 EFT Tapping Statements for Being Extraordinary!
100 EFT Tapping Statements for Fear of Computers
100 EFT Tapping Statements for Feeling Deserving
100 EFT Tapping Statements for Feeling Fulfilled
200 EFT Tapping Statements for Conflict
200 EFT Tapping Statements for Healing a Broken Heart
200 EFT Tapping Statements for Knowing God
200 EFT Tapping Statements for Positive Thinking vs
Positive Avoidance
200 EFT Tapping Statements for Procrastination
200 EFT Tapping Statements for PTSD
200 EFT Tapping Statements for Sex

200 EFT Tapping Statements for Wealth
240 EFT Tapping Statements for Fear
300 EFT Tapping Statements for Healing the Self
300 EFT Tapping Statements for Dealing with Obnoxious People
300 EFT Tapping Statements for Intuition
300 EFT Tapping Statements for Self-defeating Behaviors, Victim, Self-pity
340 EFT Tapping Statements for Healing From the Loss of a Loved One
400 EFT Tapping Statements for Being a Champion
400 EFT Tapping Statements for Being Empowered and Successful
400 EFT Tapping Statements for Dealing with Emotions
400 EFT Tapping Statements for Dreams to Reality
400 EFT Tapping Statements for My Thyroid Story
500 EFT Tapping Statements for Moving Out of Survival
700 EFT Tapping Statements for Weight, Emotional Eating, and Food Cravings
All Things EFT Tapping Manual
Emotional Significance of Human Body Parts
Muscle Testing – Obstacles and Helpful Hints

EFT TAPPING STATEMENTS FOR:
A Broken Heart, Abandonment, Anger, Depression, Grief, Emotional Healing
Anxiety, Fear, Anger, Self Pity, Change
Champion, Success, Personal Power, Self Confidence, Leader/Role Model
Prosperity, Survival, Courage, Personal Power, Success
PTSD, Disempowered, Survival, Fear, Anger
Weight & Food Cravings, Anger, Grief, Not Good Enough, Failure

Made in United States
Troutdale, OR
05/10/2024

19801546R00066